MY TRIALS

MY TRIALS

Living Life with Sugar Diabetes

ETHEREAL T. HENRY JR.

iUniverse, Inc.
Bloomington

My Trials
Living Life with Sugar Diabetes

iUniverse books may be ordered through booksellers or by contacting:

iUniverse
1663 Liberty Drive
Bloomington, IN 47403
www.iuniverse.com
1-800-Authors (1-800-288-4677)

ISBN: 978-1-4620-7130-2 (sc)
ISBN: 978-1-4620-7131-9 (ebk)

Printed in the United States of America

iUniverse rev. date: 06/26/2012

This has been a really hard time for me since my body has stopped making insulin. I used to have to worry about low blood sugar; I still have to worry about that happening. Let's talk about insulin: I have to take Lantus, Novolog, and Symlin. Let's talk about food: It has been very hard for me to eat. I have to worry about my sugar getting very high. I love fruits, but I have to watch myself because fruits make my blood sugar run high. I have to watch the food that I eat all of the time.

ETHEREAL HENRY JR.

Contents

Why Did I Want to Write This Book?

I wrote this book to share helpful information about sugar diabetes. This information comes from me, because I have lived it. A lot of this information you can't get from a doctor or a diabetes expert. I have lived it; you know exactly what I'm talking about. I am writing to share my good, my bad, my ups, and my downs of dealing with this disease. Blood testing is the most important element of living with this disease. It determines everything—insulin usage, medication dosage, food intake, and physical activity. I wrote this book to help you live your life in a positive manner. Every time I walk, my leg hurts from living with sugar diabetes. I think about my leg all the time because it hurts. So whatever I can do to make anybody's life better, I'll do it. If I can help someone with words, I'll do it. I'm writing this book because I have something important to say. This book was written to give everyone hope. You can live a successful life with this disease; there are just a lot of things you have to do to live successfully. Put blood testing at the top of the list of things you need to do to obtain success. Living with this disease since April 1983 has not been easy. One thing you have to do is forget about what happened yesterday; you cannot change it. So all our focus should be on today. Doing what you are asked to do in this book will surely give you what you need to be happy. Keeping A1c under control is our main goal. Being a type 1 diabetic has been no picnic, but if we come up with a plan with help from our doctors, we can make it. Try to make all doctor appointments; reschedule if you have to. You must put doctor appointments, having blood drawn, and any test that needs to be run at the top of your to-do list each day.

I'm so happy that I found a way to cope with this disease. The way I cope with this disease is with blood testing. Life is 80 percent mental and 20 percent physical. Why would I say that? Everything about life is mental; the mental controls the physical. In blood testing, at least there is hope. It's best to try to be happy in life. Blood testing can help me be happy; it gives me hope. The funny thing about this disease is that while I'm writing this, I'm living it. Whatever happened yesterday I cannot change. I have to focus on today. I wrote this book to tell about a lifestyle. I did not choose this lifestyle, but I'm willing to accept it. There is nothing I can do to change it, so it's better to accept it. I'm suffering from a chronic medical condition, insulin-dependant sugar diabetes. The reason this book was written was to reduce or eliminate diabetic complications. I have to discuss the good and the bad things that are going to happen to you. Even if you are using an insulin pump, some of this information can help you. I will just admit that I cannot use an insulin pump, because I will not eat right. This does not mean that using an insulin pump is not good. It is a great machine to use.

The insulin pump constantly puts insulin in your body. You have to do the right things to use this machine. It just will not work for me. Whatever works for you, do it. You need to concentrate on blood testing no matter what system you are using. This book was written to help you live your life in a positive manner when dealing with this disease. We have to become educated about this disease. We must learn something new every day. I did not write this book to tell you what you should or should not do. I wrote it just to share information that can help you live your life in a positive manner. I have learned a lot about sugar diabetes over the years by reading, studying, and listening. That's right—listening. You can obtain a lot of useful information in life by listening and not talking. I wrote this book to tell a story: my story as a type 1 diabetic. Over the years, I have often had low blood sugar as a result of trying to keep my A1c under control. That is the price we pay for trying to maintain good control.

I wrote this book to encourage anybody who has this disease to feel good about him- or herself. It's all about being happy. It's easy to say and not to do. Diabetes mellitus type 1 is what we are dealing with here. Sugar diabetes means the same thing as that Latin term. I wrote this book because God and his son, Jesus, have blessed me over the years. Nobody knows what I'm going through or what I have gone through while coping with this disease over the years. Everyone with this disease goes through trials and tribulations, but with God's help, we can make it. Every day of living with this disease has been quite an experience. My way of living has changed a lot, with all the blood tests I have to take and the need to watch my physical activity and food intake. Your lifestyle will certainly change when you have this disease. The problems

I have had over the years have come from being an insulin-dependent diabetic. Just to name a few of these problems, I've had low blood sugar, high blood sugar, trouble sleeping, restrictions on operating motor vehicles, and difficulty working. The reason I wrote this book was to tell you about a plan I have been using since I was first diagnosed with the disease in April 1983.

The Beginning

This all started in April 1983. I knew I had been getting up at night to use the bathroom quite a bit. I decided to attend a health fair that was being held in St. Louis, Missouri. They were checking for high blood pressure and for sugar diabetes. There was no charge for the tests. They told me that my blood sugar was over 250 mg/dL. A nurse told me that I was not to move out of the chair was sitting in. I was told to call the American Diabetes Association and make an appointment to see a doctor. I found a doctor named Muhammad A. Nyazee, a gastroenterologist at the Washington University School of Medicine in St. Louis. When I went to the doctor, they ran a fasting blood test, and it came back very high—again over 250 mg/dL. My next trip was an extended stay in the hospital. While I was in the hospital, I was taught how to give myself insulin injections. I stayed in the hospital a total of two weeks. I was taught how to test my urine. It seemed as if all the blood had been pumped out of my body. Every day, I'm living with the new blood.

My blood-sugar levels constantly change. Because of this, my life will never be the same. I'm seeing the same eye doctor that I began with in 1983. His name is Dr. Ramula Samudrula. When I was released from the hospital, I started using NPH insulin and regular insulin. At this time, I was working swing shift. It was not easy. Can you imagine how it felt when I was asleep and the insulin peaked out? The NPH insulin was strongest about eight hours after injection. What if I was working twelve hours or a double shift? This is why I call this the new blood. I used to have trouble all the time at work. Late at night was an especially bad time for me. I did find out an important fact: control of my blood sugar will affect how long I live and also affects how I see myself as an asset to society. When I was released, I was controlling my blood sugar with urine tests. About two years later, blood-glucose meters hit the market.

I've been using them ever since. I had to make adjustments to my life and at my job, because I worked a factory job. I was diagnosed with type 1 sugar diabetes. My body was not making any insulin. I started out taking NPH insulin and regular insulin. Regular insulin is a short-acting insulin. The NPH insulin peaked about eight hours after injection. I worked a swing shift at that time, and it was not easy. Sleeping, working, and controlling my blood sugar was not an easy task. But I did it for years, because I had to make a living. I could not draw disability just because of low blood sugar. Having to live with this disease has been quite a journey for me, but I will survive.

Insulin Usage

When I was released from the hospital in May 1983, I was using NPH and regular insulin. It was not easy working swing shift, sleeping, and controlling my blood sugar. I made it, and now I have a story to tell. The NPH used to peak about eight hours after injection. Imagine getting off work in the morning and going to sleep. While you are sleep, the insulin that is in your body somehow gets stronger. I'm not using NPH insulin now; I'm using another long-acting insulin that doesn't peak in the same way. Soon after I was released from the hospital in January 2011 (I was there to treat a burned foot), I changed my insulin usage. For all the years that I had been using long-acting insulin, I had used the sliding scale. The problem was that I used to increase my long-acting insulin dosage three or more units at a time. My doctor let me make all my insulin dosage decisions. He would give me medical advice or suggestions if I asked him. When I visited him, he asked me how much insulin I was taking. The sliding scale is when you increase or decrease your long-acting insulin dosage depending on your blood-sugar levels are.

After an accident in which I burned my foot, I decided to put the sliding scale to bed for good. On the sliding scale, you never know when your body is going to require more or less insulin. I'm not saying the sliding scale is not good at all, but it's not for me anymore. The years of having low blood sugar due to the sliding scale were too much for me. I have to fault myself, because I'm the one who gave the injections. Since I was released from the hospital in January 2011, I only decrease or increase the long-acting insulin by one unit at a time. When you increase your long-acting insulin by three or more units, the only way to tell that you don't need that dosage anymore is through blood tests or low blood sugar. When I drive a car or leave the house in someone else's car, it's a good idea to take a blood-testing machine with me. Keep a blood testing machine with you at all times. Keep extra insulin in the refrigerator at work or at home. If there is a blizzard, flood, or earthquake, you don't want to get stuck with no medication. How much regular insulin should I take at a time? How your body handles the insulin on a particular day depends on a lot of things. Do not increase your long-acting insulin more than one unit at a time, no matter how high your blood is running or has been running; it's too dangerous. Smaller changes will create fewer problems for you to deal with.

When I was in the hospital, I talked to a nurse who was treating me. She gave me a good suggestion. She said maybe I should take my oral diabetes medication at 5:00 p.m. instead of 9:00 p.m. This way, it won't be overly strong late at night when I'm sleeping. One time, I took thirty-two units of long-acting insulin before bedtime and went to sleep. I woke up and couldn't remember whether I had taken a dose earlier. So I gave myself another shot of long-acting insulin. I had a difficult night and part of the next day. I took thirty-two units of long-acting insulin by mistake. These are the kinds of mistakes insulin users will make when their bodies are not handling the insulin very well (are rejecting it). Don't panic and increase your dosage of long-acting insulin. Decrease your food intake and use regular insulin to control out-of-control blood sugar. Just don't take too much regular insulin. You never know when your body is going to change. Blood test often during this period. Even if your blood sugar has been running a little high, don't be tempted to take too much regular insulin.

Your body usually doesn't go on rejecting insulin for more than seven days. If it does, then you have to consider increasing your long-acting insulin dosage. If you do, increase it by only one unit at a time. You have to monitor your blood tests to determine when your body is close to normal. You are now dealing with the new blood, so your blood-sugar levels will be unstable from now on. You have to watch closely how much regular insulin you take and when you take it. Before you lie down to rest a little or go to sleep is not a good time to take any regular insulin.

Insulin is my life blood. I need it to survive. Since my body is not making insulin anymore, I have to inject it. Sometimes, I have to inject more than one or two units of regular insulin. I have to determine how my body is handling the insulin that day. That's why blood testing is so important to insulin usage. I'm not in agreement with making big changes in your long-acting insulin dosage. That's what I used to do—raise my dosage of long-acting insulin three, four, or five units at a time while monitoring my blood tests. All this was before I burned my foot in the shower. I recommend raising or lowering it only one unit at a time because of the problems I have had with insulin use. At times I have taken too much insulin, sometimes by accident. And boy I paid for it with hypoglycemia, which is low blood sugar.

Food Intake

We need to be educated about food choices concerning our bodies. The best ways to do this are to read and study. Read about how healthy foods affect and help your body. Sometimes, when your blood sugar is between 120 mg/dL and 155mg/dL, you can't force yourself to eat some food. This is when your body does not need a lot of food intake. Don't take a lot of regular insulin and force yourself to eat. If you do eat some food, eat a small amount and closely monitor your blood sugar. As you can see, I'm always talking about blood testing. This is the most important element of managing sugar diabetes. When your blood sugar is between these levels you need to control how much you eat. I'm not saying starve yourself to death; it's all about control. During these times, control the amount of food you eat by monitoring your blood sugar. You can help control your weight by doing this. It's a good idea to eat more fruits and vegetables. I'm not telling you to eat less meat. You must have the correct balance to keep your blood pressure and cholesterol under control. This is very important to a person who has insulin-dependent diabetes. Eating more fruits and vegetables will solve that problem.

Some days, I have a difficult time eating, because my blood-sugar levels are at or near a normal 120 mg/dL to 165 mg/dL. It's hard to eat much when you are in this range most of the day. It's kind of hard to eat when you wake up in the morning and your blood sugar is 145mg/dL. On days like this, you just can't eat a lot of food. What do you do when your blood sugar is 150mg/dL and you are hungry? Nothing. What will you do when you wake up in the morning and your blood sugar is 250 mg/dL and you are hungry? Don't eat anything; use regular insulin to bring it down. Test your blood sugar often. Don't increase your long-acting insulin right away. What do you do when your blood sugar is 260 mg/dL, you take some regular insulin to bring it down, and it goes up even higher? This is a good question. It seems as if your body is rejecting the insulin. Your body rejecting the insulin really helps you control your weight. You must control your food intake during these stressful times. The eating of fruits and vegetables has an enormous effect on my entire body. These foods contain fiber, and fiber in food is very important. Fiber retains water before waste is removed from the body. Add a lot of fruits, vegetables, and cereals that contain fiber to your diet. Eating correctly can help your body with everything—blood-sugar control, waste elimination, cholesterol, blood pressure, and many other things. Proper food intake helps with everything concerning your body. If you drink 2 percent milk and eat cereal with sliced fruit, everything will work well for you. Drink diet soda if you want it. Drink regular soda only if your blood sugar is low. You don't need to drink any diet orange juice or eat any sugar-free candy. Some people will give you these things because of their lack of education about sugar diabetes. I need the sugar; foods that don't contain sugar do me no good. The amount of food I eat is actually based on my blood-sugar levels. Sometimes I have to eat less because of the numbers. I can't just wake up and say I'm going to eat at the smorgasbord today. I have to do a lot of thinking and planning. We need to start telling people to eat some type of fruit or vegetable every time they eat meat. This will help control cholesterol and blood pressure. My job is to promote healthy eating, so of course I have to practice what I preach. Try substituting some other spice for salt on your food. Any whole-grain food low in cholesterol, saturated fat, and total fat can really help you.

My blood-sugar readings determine how much food I can eat. Using this method really helps with weight control. I'm not going to increase the long-acting insulin so that I can eat more. I might have to take a little more regular insulin if I'm going to a picnic or out to dinner. I have to do a lot of blood testing and planning. When you eat vegetables, don't get into the habit of putting butter or margarine on them every time. Try steaming or boiling them sometimes; it's healthier for you. Sometimes late at night, we eat sweet foods we shouldn't eat because of the fear of low blood sugar. If you can't eat vegetables when you're eating meat, try eating some fruit as a substitute.

Fiber is good for us. Food that contains fiber has moisture in it when it's eliminated from the body. This can help us from having or getting hemorrhoids. The name *sugar diabetes* means the same thing as the scientific term *diabetes mellitus*. It means that your body has an insufficient production of insulin. Type 1 diabetes is controlled with medication and/or insulin. Type 2 is controlled by medication only.

Blood-Sugar Control
and Body Changes

One day I was attending a morning function. After an hour and a half I went to my car to check my blood sugar. My blood sugar was 13mg/dL; the next word I uttered was yikes! I brought it up quickly. I checked it again after another hour and a half: it had gone up to 269mg/dL. It looked like it was going to be one of those days.

If you have a refrigerator at work or school, keep some juice or regular soda in it in case of emergencies. The worst thing an insulin-dependent diabetic can do is take more than one unit of regular insulin and lie down and go to sleep. If your blood sugar is high, sometimes you have to just let it be high until you wake up. Having an insulin reaction when you are sleeping is no fun. Having a blood sugar level lower than 50mg/dL is dangerous; nothing but bad things can happen. If you take more than one unit of regular insulin, you are taking a chance and playing with fire. I'm not trying to tell you how much insulin to take: all of the information here is concerning my life.

Any regular insulin you take after 6:00 p.m. will have an effect on your body if you are sleeping or working at any time after that.

Regular insulin is usually the cause of low blood sugar and can lead to an insulin reaction. Long-acting insulin can also cause insulin reactions, but not as often as regular insulin. There is no set time for your body to reject or need less insulin; it can happen at any time. Our blood sugar tests will let us know these things. Every day can be different.

I know I haven't talked at all about high blood sugars, in the three-to-seven-hundred range. With all the blood tests I run, I don't plan on letting it stay in that range too long. Sometimes your blood sugar can just cycle up without you consuming that much; this can happen at any time. I don't know the reason why. That's why we test our blood regularly to try to keep it in the proper range. We just don't want to get to the point where we don't care what our blood sugar levels are. We must be committed to controlling our A1c in a safe range.

Keeping our A1c tests under control will help you avoid diabetic complications. That's why I feel blood testing is the most important part of sugar diabetes management. I mentioned above that the regular blood was pumped out of my body. I'm living with the new blood every day. The new blood has blood-sugar levels that constantly change. I have no idea each day how my body is going to react to insulin or oral diabetes medication.

Foot care is very important. Check your feet and between your toes every day. Trim your toenails straight across as needed. Use moisturizing cream on your feet as needed. Have foot and eye exams at least twice a year. Don't do what I did. I did not get a foot doctor until

I had had the disease for twenty-six years. I woke up one morning and my blood sugar was at 57mg/dL—ugh! That's kind of low. Sugar diabetes makes you feel really tired at times.

All through the day it was between 105mg/dL and 140mg/dL. When I ate some food during the day, it was only small amounts. I took only one or two units of regular insulin at a time, because my body was really handling the insulin well for a few days. Great! Everyone who is insulin-dependent has low blood sugar at some point. I don't really know how to control it late at night. The only thing I can tell anyone to do is to blood test if they are able. Blood testing gives a way to judge how we are doing. If we don't blood test, we don't know how our sugar diabetes management is doing. Sugar diabetes is just another name for *diabetes mellitus*, which means your body produces insufficient insulin. Whatever you do, don't take too much regular insulin when eating any food. If you take too much regular insulin, your body will let you know.

A low-blood-sugar reaction will be more severe when combined with an increase in long-acting insulin and regular insulin. Sometimes if you work the day shift, it may be difficult to wake up in the morning if your blood sugar is too low. There have been times when I have taken too much insulin by accident; sometimes it just happens. If you know you have taken too much insulin, you have to blood test your way out of the problem. The fingers on both of my hands look like I have dipped them in a bowl of black pepper. They look like this because of the many years of blood testing. I really have to be concerned about myself when I go to sleep or take a nap. Do not take more than one unit of regular insulin if you lie down with blood sugar at 180mg/dL or higher. Your body can react differently to insulin at any time. You can be above 250mg/dL, take two units of regular insulin, and fall asleep, and your blood sugar can drop extremely quickly. You have to be very careful about the way you handle this situation. Maybe taking one unit of regular insulin would be safer. It depends on how tired you are and how long you plan to sleep. There are times when your body totally rejects the insulin. Your blood sugar can drop to any number when you are asleep. There is no way to tell how fast your blood sugar will drop or what your blood-sugar number will be. It's a good idea not to take a lot of regular insulin in the evening after 6:00 p.m. It depends on how your body is handling the insulin that day. Other factors to consider include your level of physical activity and whether you are going to be doing a lot of driving.

You can tell by your high blood-sugar readings when you wake up after sleeping. It can also happen when you haven't eaten very much or anything at all. Whatever you do, don't increase your long-acting insulin more than one unit at a time. If you do, you are only asking for trouble.

Use more regular insulin for blood-sugar control during this time. You can tell when your body is not rejecting the insulin by your blood-sugar levels. During these times, we really have to watch what we eat and check our blood sugar to keep it under control.

This occurs at times when you haven't eaten anything. What do you do when your blood sugar is 155mg/dL and you are very hungry? Wait an hour and test your blood sugar again. My prescription for blood strips says to check your blood eight times a day. It's important to believe in what you are doing, and that means believing in blood testing. In the end, everything will turn out well. Low blood sugar is one of my greatest fears in life.

If you wake up between 1:00 a.m. and 6:00 a.m., test your blood sugar, and if it's under 100mg/dL, drink a cup of orange juice or eat something sweet before you go back to sleep. Low blood sugar can cause you to sleep longer. Sometimes, when your body is rejecting the insulin, your blood-sugar levels will increase. One day I tested my blood sugar at about 5:00 p.m., and it was at 134mg/dL. I checked again at 7:00 p.m., and it had increased to 305mg/dL without my eating or drinking anything. Another day, I was supposed to take someone to work at 6:15 p.m. I woke up at 5:30 a.m. and tested my blood sugar, and it was 39mg/dL. I fell right back to sleep and didn't take that person to work. When I woke up at about 8:30 a.m., water was overflowing in the bathroom sink and running on the carpet and down the stairs. It's a good thing the water didn't run into the fuse box. It didn't take long for my blood sugar to drop low. The low-blood-sugar bandit had struck again.

There is currently no cure for sugar diabetes; the emphasis must be put on treatment and management to avoid complications. Diabetes treatment and management techniques include weight control, blood testing, a healthy diet, and oral diabetes medication. Self blood testing is the key to maintaining a successful life. When dealing with this disease, the first thing to do is to feel good about yourself. Yes, that's what I said. Then you will have confidence in what you are doing. Believe that blood testing will reduce the chances of having diabetic complications. Believe that blood testing will be the key to living with sugar diabetes. My blood sugar is unstable. Sometimes my body rejects the insulin. This means that during certain times, my body is not using the insulin correctly. We have to blood test when our blood sugar increases on its own without any food or drink intake. Why does your blood sugar just go up? I really don't have an answer to this question. Remember that the insulin you take is foreign to the body. Sometimes, your blood sugar will just cycle up on its own during a certain time period. A normal person's blood sugar is controlled without a hitch. For a person with sugar diabetes, controlling blood sugar requires a lifetime of insulin injections and blood testing. Most of our low blood-sugar readings occur because of the injection of regular insulin. This doesn't happen all the time; sometimes long-acting insulin can also cause the problem.

Body Injuries and Sores

I have to monitor any cuts or sores I get on my lower extremities. I have to wear heavy socks or an elastic tubular bandage on both feet. The ends of both feet on the socks have to be sewed up, and they have to extend at least halfway up the leg. I have to wear them when I lie down to go to sleep at night. This provides protection to my legs and feet when my blood sugar falls when I sleep. It protects my legs when they hit something—the wall, a chair, or a dresser. I have to check my toes, toenails, feet, and lower legs for injuries. As an insulin-dependent diabetic, I'm likely to have infections and slow healing. Sometimes I get injuries from my feet or legs hitting the wall or the dresser. Sometimes after getting an injury, I think to myself that maybe it would be better if I slept in a padded room. Ha ha!

I had an unbelievable car wreck in June 2008. I had just bought a brand new 2008 Hyundai Accent. About ten minutes after I drove off the lot, I drove the car into another car lot. I guess I was trying to get two deals in one day? My car looked like a crushed eggshell. It was totaled.

It's a good thing I did not end up paralyzed or have any internal injuries. Low blood sugar had struck again.

I had hypoglycemia and passed out while driving the car. This is one of the reasons I always should check my blood sugar before I start driving. I ran into a used-car lot and did $24,000 of damage to two used cars. I had only $10,000 of property-damage insurance. I was sued for $24,000. The car-lot dealer did me a favor. We settled for $14,000, and the insurance company paid $10,000 and I paid $4,000. I learned a life-changing lesson. Anyone who has insulin-dependent sugar diabetes who drives a car should have the maximum property-damage insurance on any vehicles they drive. I suffered a broken leg in the accident. The x-rays still look bad to me. They put a bar and two pins in my left leg. I have pain in my leg all the time. I'm not able to work. In Sept 2009, I had a low-blood-sugar reaction late at night while sleeping. When I woke up, blood was everywhere. I had hit my right Achilles tendon on the metal bed frame. I ended up with a diabetic ulcer on my right leg. I put some triple-antibiotic ointment on it. It would not heal.

I went to a foot doctor for the first time in my life. He did a graft-jacket surgery on my Achilles tendon, and it was a success. The skin that was used is made from donated human skin, which undergoes a process that removes the epidermis and dermal cells. In Jan 2011, I took a nap in the morning. When I woke up, I was standing in the shower, and hot water was running on my right foot. The tub was about a third of the way filled up. Low blood sugar had struck again. I put triple-antibiotic pain ointment on my foot as it blistered up. I went to the foot doctor two days later, and he put me in the hospital immediately. I was diagnosed with a third-degree burn and other blisters on my right foot. I was put on an IV and antibiotics to help heal and prevent infection. The funny thing about this is that when I went to the foot doctor, he told me, "Mr. Henry, you have go check into the hospital right now." I thought that was pretty funny. I kid him about what he said to me sometimes.

I stayed in the hospital for seven days. After three weeks of home health care, my foot finally healed. One day when I had low blood sugar late at night, I hit my hand on something and skinned my knuckles. One morning, I had low blood sugar and was given some juice. The next day, half the white of one of my eyes was dark red. It happened because of low blood sugar. This is why we have to set a certain time—in my case, it's 6:00 p.m.—after which we don't take any more regular insulin. If it's in your body, it will affect you immediately or later when you are sleeping. The only time we should take regular insulin in the evening is when our blood sugar is running a little high. This is why we should test our blood sugar constantly. Everything is determined by blood tests—how much food we eat and how much insulin we take. I don't know how much food I should eat or how much insulin I should take, but my body does. Sometimes when I hit my knuckles I end up with painful sores on them. There are some mornings when I wake with a big knot on my forehead. I also sometimes have sores that can happen anywhere on my body. Why? It's all because of low blood sugar! Don't take any regular insulin after 6:00 p.m. unless you have to in order to eat some food or because you have a high blood-sugar level. This will have to be determined by the blood tests you take. Sometimes, the regular insulin you take after 6:00 p.m. will affect your body late at night while you sleep. That can cause you to have more injuries and sores. Taking less insulin will require you to eat less food; this is a way to help you control your weight.

This was not an easy chapter to write. Yes, life has been sore at times for me, but I always heal. I have to put medicine and bandages on some sores that I get on my body. I do this to help prevent them from becoming infected. Some days I wake up, have sores, and don't remember how I got them. The sores, cuts, and bruises are just problems that come with having sugar diabetes.

But remember: even though there are complications like these, by maintaining good control of our A1c over the years, we can delay or not have to deal with some of the complications associated with this disease. Though the cuts, sores, and bruises are bad, I would rather deal with them than the early kidney machine use or the early loss of a limb (leg) caused by bad A1c control. Yes, I'm speaking about good control and declaring it to be a way to victory. You can do it!

Blood Testing

We must test our blood sugar all the time, even when we don't feel like it. It could be late at night or early in the morning. Whenever you wake up, test your blood sugar. This is my favorite chapter in the book. Why? Because I would not be writing this if it weren't for blood testing. Blood testing is what keeps me living. Blood testing has no certain time. Whatever time you test your blood is good. This is also my favorite chapter because I believe that blood testing is the most important part of diabetes management. If you have a conversation with me about sugar diabetes, soon blood testing will come up. My blood-sugar level can even affect my personality and how I act. It can make you act violent. It can make you not react at all when you probably should. This is why we must test our blood sugar all the time. Low blood sugar can make you say a lot of things you will be sorry about later. It is a good idea to test your blood sugar before you begin to drive. I check my blood sugar while I'm driving; I do not recommend doing that. It only takes me about ten seconds. I am not a doctor, and I'm not saying you should do this. If I'm in the middle of traffic and I start sweating or can feel that I have low blood sugar, I have to test myself while driving.

Don't forget that your body can change. Different foods can have different effects on your blood sugar. Sometimes if you forget to take any medication or insulin, it can cause your blood sugar to rise. I have done this many times. If you take any medication, don't go more than one day without taking it. If you do, it can cause your numbers to rise, which is very dangerous. If you are using the sliding scale to control your blood sugar, increase or decrease the dosage by only one unit at a time. One morning when I woke up my blood-sugar level was 156mg/dL, which is acceptable. During the day, my blood sugar stayed close to 125mg/dL. I didn't eat too much that day. Sometimes you can tell if your blood sugar is high or low from your body temperature. When your body feels cold, your blood sugar is usually low. One day I woke up at 2:10 a.m. and tested my blood sugar, and it was 165mg/dL. Since my tests had been running a little high the past three days, I took one unit of regular insulin and went back to sleep. I woke up at 6:00 a.m., and my blood sugar had dropped to 68mg/dL. Now that is really unstable. Having type 1 sugar diabetes gives you the job of keeping your A1c under control. From the time you start taking insulin, it turns into a lifetime job. Any time I wake up to use the restroom late at night, it is a good idea to run a blood test. When I first was diagnosed with sugar diabetes in April 1983, I started out just doing urine tests and logging the date, time, and blood-sugar level. A couple of years later, everyone started blood and A1c testing. Technology has changed so much that you don't have to write your readings down anymore. You can put them on your computer and have access to them.

The A1c test is the most important blood test that we take. The main reason I have suffered from many low-blood-sugar readings over the years is a result of my attempts to try to keep my blood sugar levels under control. The A1c test is a three-month average of your blood sugars. Put blood testing at the top of the list as part of your diabetes management. What is the first thing you should do when you wake up in the morning?

Test your blood sugar. It would be a good idea to test your blood before every time you are going to operate a motor vehicle. If it's low, bring it up to a safe range before you start driving. If I have to attend a meeting or go to an appointment, most of the time I test my blood before I go in. Keep some hard candy with you at all times. If I have a long way to walk, I will put my blood testing machine and insulin in my pocket. If I have to use either of them, I can always go to the men's restroom.

Driving

Driving an automobile can be quite an adventure at times. We have to keep our blood sugar under control while driving. I check my blood sugar while driving; it's not that much of a distraction. I might be in traffic and need to check my blood right away. It takes less than ten seconds. I don't have time to pull over if I'm on an interstate highway or on a very busy street. I'm not suggesting you test your blood sugar while driving; that's your decision. But I have to do what I have to do in order to be able to drive. It works for me, but maybe it would not work for anyone else. Doctors, nurses, and book editors might disagree. Most of these people have never had to run any kind of blood test on themselves ever. It would be interesting to learn if any of these people have a sense of humor.

I have a few questions to ask them: Have you ever had low blood sugar while driving and run off of the road as a result? Have you ever been asleep in bed and couldn't wake up because of low blood sugar? The answer to both of these questions is most likely no. This is why I test my blood whenever and wherever I can.

Blood testing is very important to me; it's the most important part of my diabetes management. I learned the hard way that you have to test your blood while you drive sometimes. I don't worry about who agrees or disagrees; it's easy to have an opinion about something that doesn't involve you. When an issue directly involves you, your way of thinking will be much different.

Now, before I begin driving, I always test my blood. Whenever you start driving, the first thing you should do is check your blood sugar. If you don't, you may have to pay a price for it later. Try to keep your blood sugar at or above 100mg/dL any time you are driving. Your activities have a lot to do with your blood-sugar levels while you are driving. If you are driving two hundred or more miles, it is a good idea to keep your blood sugar at or above 100 mg/dL. When you get it in this range, check it every hour while you are driving. Your blood sugar can drop really fast at any time. This is where blood testing comes into play. Blood-sugar testing is like drinking water; it is something you have to do all the time. If your blood sugar drops rapidly while you are driving, it can be quite an experience. You can lose all sense of judgment and thought. You can start driving erratically or you can have a serious car wreck. I know it has happened to me. If you are an insured driver of a motor vehicle, you should consider increasing the property damage insurance to $25,000. You heard it first right here, so spread the word.

Anybody who is an insulin-dependent diabetic should have $25,000 of property damage insurance. You never know what can happen. It's not going to cost you that much more money, and boy is it worth it. Before you put that key in the ignition, don't forget to test your blood sugar. If you are driving and for some reason you can't test your blood sugar, it would be a good idea to put a couple pieces of candy in your mouth. Do this if you are unsure what your blood-sugar level is. It's better to be safe than sorry. It's a good idea to keep some juice, candy, or some other type of food in the car that will raise your blood sugar quickly. Maintain and monitor blood sugar at all times while driving. Do this to prevent driving down a one-way street or going the wrong way on an interstate highway. This can be disastrous if it happens. With sugar diabetes, anything can happen. Always know what your blood-sugar level is while you are driving. Don't assume, guess, or think anything. It doesn't take that long to run a blood test while you are driving and isn't much of a distraction. Everyone might not agree, so I'm not saying you absolutely should test your blood sugar while driving, but sometimes it may be the less risky option. Most people who don't have sugar diabetes will disagree with me, but most people who disagree have never learned how to take a blood test. I don't need to pull over every time I have to run a blood test. If I had to do that every time I took a blood test, life would be very boring. I'm trying to do whatever I can to survive. If you have had lupus for twenty years, I'm not going to tell you what you should or shouldn't do, because I haven't had it and it wouldn't be fair of me.

If you don't check your blood sugar before you start driving, bad things can happen. When I had the car wreck in June 2008, it happened because of low blood sugar and lack of blood testing. In May 2011, I left home early in the morning to go to the store. Of course, I didn't check my blood sugar. I ran into the back of a car. They called the police, and the paramedics came. The paramedics said my blood sugar was 40mg/dL. The paramedics gave me some glucose and brought my blood sugar up, so they let me drive away. I made a mistake by not checking my blood sugar before I started driving. I'm not perfect, but things like this can happen. It's very easy to get discouraged by what happens to you in life. Test your blood and know what your numbers are; blood testing would have solved this problem. My blood sugar was so low that I didn't think to test my blood sugar. Here is a new policy to live by: don't test, don't drive. I have blamed myself for any accident I had that was caused by low blood sugar. I don't suggest that everyone test their blood sugar while driving. I know it works for me. It only takes me about ten seconds. I'm not a doctor, and you don't have to do what I'm doing. This is a thought for anyone who drives and is insulin dependent. Anyone who has passed out while driving might agree with me. It's not a distraction for me, but I'm not suggesting that you try it.

Don't leave home without your blood-testing machine and insulin, even if you are riding with someone else. When I passed out while driving in June 2008, it happened without warning. I knew I had taken some regular insulin and would be driving. It's a good thing that I didn't make it back to I-70 before passing out. I would have been on the highway and driving at a higher speed. I probably wouldn't be writing this book today. If only I had blood tested myself! It seems as if driving and blood testing were not really important to me. Now all that has changed, because today I will not attempt to drive without blood testing. You have to watch yourself sometimes, because if your blood sugar gets too low, you can forget where you parked your car. Always carry an extra set of keys in case you lock your keys in the car or lose them.

Working

I worked swing shift from 1983 to 1999. I had to do a lot of blood testing just to make it during that time. I started out using regular insulin and NPH insulin. At that time, I was taking the NPH at about 7:00 a.m., and it peaked out around 3:00 p.m. I worked a factory job, and it was not easy. It was really difficult to work all three shifts. Sometimes I would have to work twelve or sixteen hours. Being an insulin-dependent diabetic can be a very touchy situation. If you work a physically demanding job (or even an easy job), you have to work at handling this disease. You have to check your blood sugar often. I can't tell you how often to check your blood sugar; that is something you have to work out for yourself. But it should probably be more than three times in an eight-to-sixteen-hour work day. You should have access to a blood-testing machine at your job. We have to do blood testing as our jobs permit so that it doesn't become a distraction to our work groups. Keep some extra blood strips, insulin, and your normal medication with you; you never know when you will be stuck at work. Just think how hard it was working in a factory operating machinery and driving pay loaders and fork lifts. I really had to keep a close watch on my blood sugar all the time, and it wasn't easy.

While at work is not a time to take a lot of regular insulin, no matter how your readings are running. Keep some hard candy on you at all times. I used to think I was a problem to people I worked with because of sugar diabetes. Even though I was testing myself at work, there was the chance for the occasional low-blood-sugar reaction. If you work or go to school, let the people in charge know about your health situation and educate them if you can. The same thing applies to coworkers, bosses, and security. When you are at work, you should blood test yourself as often as your work permits. Try not to overexert yourself, depending on the type of work you do. The job I had when I had the terrible car wreck in 2008 required me to move rental cars. Sometimes I moved them on the lot or to other lots, and sometimes I moved them out of town. I had to check my blood sugar all the time while I was driving. It was not easy, but here I am, still living and writing a book. I have so much to be thankful for—the people on my jobs who knew what I was dealing with and all the supervisors I have ever worked for.

Paramedic Visits

During my twenty-eight years of having sugar diabetes, I have had many visits from the paramedics. It is not easy for me to write this chapter. Any time you put insulin in your body, there is a chance of having a bad reaction. A reaction is an action in response to an agent, influence, or stimulus; a chemical change. If the police and paramedics come, they come to help you. The reason they usually come is low blood sugar. It is good to wear a necklace or bracelet. It should inform the paramedics that you have sugar diabetes and list any other medication you take. A card in your wallet would be good too. It could have independent information or a number to call to get diabetic information. I'm not going to get into the details of the paramedic visits. I really have tried hard all of these years to keep my blood sugar under control. Trying to keep it under control is probably why I've had a lot of low blood sugar many times over the course of my life. I have found that my blood sugar is very unstable. My A1c is high, I can't bring it down, or it runs low all the time. My grandmother always told me, "Can't ain't in the book." If I ever wake up and see paramedics, I say, "Good, I'm still living."

One of the great secrets of success is failure. We have to take risks again and again. Do this in order to find the winning combination. This may be difficult for people who try nothing unless it looks like it will be a winner. Failure makes us enjoy success. A paramedic visit can be viewed as a failure. But the knowledge we get from it can be viewed as a success. Don't be embarrassed by a paramedic visit; it's just one of the things in life you can't control. If you have sugar diabetes, sometimes things like this are going to happen. If you have high A1c numbers, you probably don't know what a low-blood-sugar reaction is and have never had one that required paramedics. If you are walking around every day with blood-sugar levels between 250mg/dL and 500mg/dL or even higher, that is not good. If your numbers are in that range, you can't be doing a lot of blood testing.

Sleeping

Sleeping can be a very difficult struggle for a Type 1 diabetic. We cannot control our blood sugar when we are sleeping, or even when we are taking a catnap.

We don't know what our blood sugar levels are during sleep: high, low, or normal? Whenever we plan to sleep, we need to check our blood sugar, if possible, before we go to sleep and when we wake up. Time doesn't matter; there is no set time for checking your blood sugar. If your blood sugar drops low while you are sleeping, at times you will do a lot of sweating. If your blood sugar is low, you can wake up without knowing what day or time it is, along with other things. You can sleep through alarms, miss appointments, and be late for work or school. If you don't wake up on time or you sleep through an alarm, this was probably because of low blood sugar. That is why it's sometimes best to use two alarm clocks, though sometimes that doesn't work. If you wake up at any time late at night to use the bathroom, it is a good idea to check your blood sugar to see were your level is.

One of my greatest fears is that my blood sugar will drop down too low while I'm sleeping. I have no way to control the circumstances when that happens. That can be a reason you wake up sometimes with sores on your body. Sometimes, if you are sleeping and your blood sugar gets low, you can have nightmares.

The Bad

Most of my worst experiences with this disease have been related to low blood sugar. I have trouble waking up in the morning because of low blood sugar. Sometimes I have needed to go to work or to an appointment but couldn't wake up. There is a way to help solve this problem. I have at least two alarms set at two different times to wake me up. I have had many visits from the paramedics. It's just something that happens to people who have sugar diabetes. I was being treated for low blood sugar. I have had a few holes in the wall and a torn shower curtain from having low blood sugar. I have had many cuts on my legs and sores on my feet and forehead from low blood sugar. My feet or legs sometimes hit the wall or the dresser, causing injuries. This is not easy for me to write about. You are what your blood-sugar level is. If it drops too low and you are still conscious, it can affect your personality. It can also affect decisions you make. In June 2008 I had a day off from my job, so I went to St. Charles, Missouri, and purchased a brand-new 2008 Hyundai Accent.

Before I left home, I checked my blood sugar, and it was between 230mg/dL and 245mg/dL. Then I took two units of regular insulin. I had to go over to Illinois on Route 3, not far from St. Louis, to the credit union. When I returned to the dealership, we completed the deal for the new car. I left the dealership, and I was so excited about my new car that I didn't even think about checking my blood sugar. As I was driving on one of the outer roads off I-70 in St. Charles, I passed out while driving because of low blood sugar. Some witnesses said that I was driving erratically before the accident, but I don't remember. I crashed into a used-car-dealership lot. I suffered a broken leg, and my new car was totaled. I did damage to two cars on the lot that ended totaling $24,000 in property damage. This is the reason I wrote above that a person with insulin-dependent diabetes should have $25,000 of property damage insurance. If you run into a house, apartment, or anything else of great value, the damage could be astronomical. I had $10,000 of property damage insurance, so the dealership sued me for $24,000. We settled the case. The insurance company paid $10,000. The dealership dropped $10,000, and I had to pay $4,000. I stayed in the hospital for seven days. I had a broken left leg. They had to put a bar and two pins in my leg. I had soreness and pain for about a month from my waist to my neck. The x-rays for my leg still don't look good. It took about four months before I finally started walking again. When I first broke my leg, I could only go three places with a walker—the bathroom, my bed, and the sofa. I have had pain in my leg every day since the accident. It took me about four months before I finally started walking again. I have not worked since the accident.

In September of 2009, I had low blood sugar late at night. I ended up hitting my right Achilles tendon on the steel bed frame. I had a diabetic ulcer. The injury was pretty bad. Since it was on the lower part of my body where there is less blood, the injury would not heal. I put triple-antibiotic ointment on it, and it didn't work. I had never had a foot doctor during all my years of having sugar diabetes. I chose Dr. Zachary J. Newland in Louis, Missouri. He gave me out-patient surgery using a graft jacket, a treatment for diabetic foot ulcers with chronic, nonhealing wounds. My insurance company would not pay for the operation. The insurance company said it would be better to have an amputation. Their review board said the operation was experimental at best. Dr. Newland did the operation. After implantation, the body's natural repair process revascularizes and repopulates the graft-jacket matrix. It uses cells that allow the body to convert the graft-jacket matrix into living skin tissue. This means that the body can use the graft-jacket matrix as it repairs itself. It is made from donated human skin, which undergoes a process that removes the epidermis and dermal cells. The operation was a success. I was so thankful, because before the procedure, it would not heal. My insurance company told me that their review board would not authorize the operation. I was really shocked. They told me that having an amputation would not be considered a bad thing. My doctor told me not to worry about it and that he would take care of it. Now isn't that really caring for another human being? That's why I wrote this book—to try to help someone in some way with knowledge or just encouragement. When living with sugar diabetes, there's something new all the time. What I mean is that there are a lot of bad things that happen to you when you are dealing with sugar diabetes. So many bad things have happened to me that I can't mention them all.

In January of 2011, I took a nap one day at 11:00 a.m. When I woke up, I was standing in the bathtub. Hot water had been running on my right foot, and the tub was a third of the way full. I was suffering from low blood sugar. I put some triple-antibiotic ointment on it. I had an appointment with my regular doctor, Dr. A. Nyazee, but I didn't say anything about it to him, because I didn't think it was that bad. The next day, my foot started to develop blisters from the burn. I could still walk, but my toes began to swell up. This happened on a Monday. On Wednesday, I went to my foot doctor, Dr Zachary J. Newland. Sometimes when I see him now, I kid him about what he said to me that day. "Mr. Henry, you need to go and check into the hospital right now." I checked into De Paul Hospital that same day. I was found to have a third-degree burn on the top of my right foot. I also had blisters on other parts of my foot. I was treated with Silvadene cream, antibiotic pills, and IVs. This was done to help prevent infection. I stayed in the hospital for seven days. The blisters and the burn wound healed due to great medical care. After I was released from the hospital, I started keeping my long-acting insulin at a consistent dosage. I stopped making large increases of three to five units based on my blood test readings. I started increasing or decreasing the long-acting insulin by just one unit at a time. I know at times my body is going to reject the insulin. That's when I have to eat less, blood test, and take my oral diabetes medication.

One day in May 2011, I woke up early in the morning and went to the store. I did not check my blood sugar before I got into the car to drive. I rear-ended a car, and the woman driving it called the police. After that, the next thing I can remember is being in the ambulance. They had given me some glucose by IV. They tested my blood glucose again, and it was about 165mg/dL. They let me drive home after that.

Even if you have health insurance, the visits can get pretty expensive. I have not worked since the car accident that broke my leg. I have pain in my leg every day. The leg has a bar and two pins in it. That leg is bigger than the other leg. I have kicked holes in the drywall while sleeping from having low blood sugar. High blood sugar over a period of years can cause damage to the brain, eyes, heart, and kidneys. That is the main reason people with diabetes must follow a blood-testing plan. The signs of sugar diabetes are blurred vision, urinating a lot, and being thirsty all the time. If you have had these problems for some time, it would be a good idea to take a blood-sugar test to see where you stand. When I was found to have sugar diabetes, I had some of these problems. One day, I woke up with low blood sugar and found that I had bitten my tongue, and blood was all over the bed. Blood was all over my pajama top and the bed.

The Good

The good things that have come out of living with sugar diabetes are many. I'm able to control my intake of food by monitoring my blood-sugar levels constantly. This helps me control my weight. It's kind of hard to eat a lot of food when your blood-sugar levels are between 125 mg/dL and 165mg/dL. This happens to me quite a bit. So at times I'm really hungry, but I can't eat a lot of food. I don't have to take a lot of regular insulin all the time just to eat more food. Right now, if I need to increase my long-acting insulin, I only do so by one unit at a time. No more three-unit or more increases at once for me. When I made large increases of long-acting insulin in the past, it usually came back to haunt me. I have been controlling blood-sugar spikes with food intake, oral medication, and regular insulin. I have been eating a lot of carrots, broccoli, and other vegetables. I also eat a lot of oranges, watermelon, strawberries, grapes, and other fruits. Having this disease has taught me what foods and how much I can eat. The new blood really has me going. Eating a lot of fruits and vegetables can really help prevent you from getting hemorrhoids. Your diet controls a lot of functions within your body. We have to control our blood-sugar levels by doing this, but it's well worth it.

Having sugar diabetes has taught me how to monitor my blood sugar, blood pressure, and cholesterol. I'm so happy that I have found a way to cope with this disease. It is with blood testing. With blood testing, at least there is hope. It's best to try to be happy in life. Blood testing can help me be happy; it gives me hope. I mention blood testing quite a bit in this book. Blood testing is the greatest good associated with having this disease. After I had my last low-blood-sugar accident, I started blood testing every time I wake up late at night and every time I drive a car.

Questions about Sugar Diabetes

1. What should I do if people call me to pick them up and take them to work, and they are in a hurry to get to work, but my blood sugar is at 49 mg/dL?

    The first thing to do is to eat or drink something to bring your blood sugar up. Don't start driving until it starts climbing. Take something to eat or drink while you are driving. Check your blood sugar while you are driving. Check it every half hour until it reaches 100 mg/dL.

2. How do I educate people about sugar diabetes?

    The first thing to do is to educate yourself. Start telling people that your pancreas is not making any insulin. Explain how your body uses insulin. You cannot do this with one conversation. It will take a while to educate people. Tell them everything that you know associated with this disease.

3. How do I keep access to my insulin and syringes when I travel?

   When you travel, always keep extra bottles of long-acting and regular insulin with you. I have dropped a bottle of insulin on a hard floor and had it break. It would be a good idea to carry extra syringes too. If you are in a car, how much you bring depends on how far you are traveling and the weather. Keep it refrigerated if you can. Wear a bracelet or some type of diabetes identification. It all depends on the number of days you will be traveling. The medicine or any type of medical device should have your name and the prescribing doctor's name on it. Don't put all the things you need in one suitcase. What will you do if the luggage is lost or goes to another city?

4. How often should I check my blood sugar?

   Check your blood sugar whenever you feel you should. There should be no set time for checking your blood sugar. When you wake up, check it. Every time you wake up at night to use the bathroom, check it.

5. My blood sugar is low all the time. What can I do about it?

   Blood testing is a must; it is something we have to do. Adjust your long-acting insulin based on your blood tests. Increase or decrease the dosage by one unit at a time. Try taking your diabetes pills at about 5:00 p.m. That way, it won't be really strong late at night. Take fewer doses of regular insulin. Blood testing is one of my favorite phrases. Regular insulin is fast-acting insulin, but it can still have an effect on you hours after an injection. Less can be more. Try taking less insulin. The less insulin you take, the more control you will have over your blood sugar.

6. What will happen to me if I don't take care of myself and don't care what happens to me?

You won't be able to live. From this day on, you need to start living life positively and not negatively. We are not trying to beat this disease; we are just trying to deal with it the best way possible. I'm using the word we, because I have to do the same thing you do. If we don't care about or take care of ourselves, only bad things can happen. We run the risk of early manifestations of diabetic complications. This will happen for sure if we neglect our bodies. This happens after years of having high blood sugar. How many years? It depends on how much we care. We have to work with our doctors to bring our A1c into the 6.0 to 7.9 range, which is acceptable. With an A1c in that range, you can live a lot of productive years.

When people see you attempting to take care of yourself, they will offer you an encouraging word, and that can help keep you operating in a positive matter. They see what you are doing and will sometimes try to help you.

It all depends on your attitude. It says a lot about your reason for living, You can ask this question over and over again: "Why did this have to happen to me?" We were born into an imperfect world. That is why everything, including our lives, is not perfect. So let us deal with this disease the best way we can. You might not believe this, but you are your own best doctor. How? By doing the things that you are supposed to do.

7. I'm overweight. How do I lose weight?

You must blood test all the time. Lower your long-acting insulin to a set number. Eat a lot of fruits and vegetables. Use small amounts of regular insulin to control blood-sugar levels. Eat smaller meals and less meat. You should see the weight start dropping off. In this case, less is more. The less insulin you use, the more weight will drop off. The more insulin you take, the more your body will crave food.

8. My cholesterol and blood pressure stay high; what can I do about it?

It's all about your diet. Eat more fruits and vegetables, and reduce your meat intake. Take your medication as prescribed, and you should see a drop in both.

9. Sometimes when I go to sleep at night, I wake up lying on the floor, and the bed is all messed up. What has happened?

What has happened is that your blood sugar got low while you were sleeping. This is just one of the problems that insulin-dependent diabetics have. There is really no way to solve this problem. We can constantly check our blood sugar and reduce the amount of regular insulin that we use.

ETHEREAL T. HENRY JR.

10. What do I do if my blood sugar is over 300mg/dL and I'm not at home?

   If you're driving, don't take too much regular insulin. At this time, take only two units of regular insulin and no more. If you are not driving, do the same thing. Dealing with unstable blood sugar can be trying. Check your blood sugar every half hour during these times. Who knows when the body is going to change? Don't take a large amount of regular insulin, because then you will have trouble with low blood sugar.

11. What if my blood sugar is high and I take some regular insulin, and in an hour it hasn't dropped or has even gone up by 40mg/dL?

   The funny thing about taking insulin is that your body never gets used to it, because it is foreign to your body. This is when you have to be patient. Keep doing the most important element of diabetes management: blood testing. In this case, it is likely that your body is rejecting the insulin at this time. Reduce your food intake. Use regular insulin carefully to bring your blood sugar under control.

12. My A1c tests run high all the time. What can I do to bring my A1c down?

   This is a good question. The first thing you have to do is a lot of blood testing. Blood test before you eat and one to two hours after eating. If you take diabetes medication, make sure you take medication at the proper times. Don't take too much regular insulin each time you are trying to control your blood-sugar levels. Watch your blood-sugar levels and control them when they cycle up on their own. Increase your long-acting insulin one unit at a time if you have to. Don't increase it more than two units total.

Epilogue

This book was written to encourage you. You can live successfully with sugar diabetes. Establish a good meal plan with good food choices so that you can eat healthfully. Count carbohydrates or use the glycemic index. With each meal, monitor fats and saturated fats, and find out how certain foods affect your blood sugar. See if you can talk to a dietitian so that you can set up a meal plan. Closely monitor your weight all the time. Education and blood testing are the keys to living a productive life. Self-assurance is an important part of this journey. Self assurance is the faith in one's own judgment or ability. You have to feel confident about yourself—starting today. The first you thing you should do when you wake up is say something good about yourself. It is very important for you to feel good about yourself when living with this disease. I could have let all the misfortunes and setbacks that I have experienced discourage me, but I chose not to. There is no way I could have made it all these years without feeling good about myself. When friends, family, or coworkers see you trying to take care of yourself, they will try to help you. You have to educate them about what they don't know about sugar diabetes. You must focus on everything positive and nothing negative. You have to forget what happened yesterday; there is no way you can change it. Don't feel sad when things don't go your way. You can make it; tell yourself that you can. This book contains a lot of information that you won't hear on the street and that nobody talks about. People will say strange things about sugar diabetes: "Call the paramedics. His or her blood sugar must be low." "He or she doesn't look right. What's wrong with him or her?" "That person must be sick." But I've got good news for you: you and I are going to have control over this disease. How? By following a vigorous blood-testing program. Don't eat more meat than fruits or vegetables. Do check your blood sugar at least four times a day. Blood testing is at the top of my list in my diabetes care. Blood testing is the most important part of diabetes care. I have learned the value of the ABCs of blood testing:

A. A1c testing,
B. blood-glucose testing, and
C. cholesterol testing.

For reference, here are some words related to this disease as well as their definitions.

1. A1c blood test: Blood sugar average over a three-month period.

2. hyperglycemia: An abnormally high level of glucose in the blood. When sustained over a

prolonged period of time, extremely high blood sugar can cause or lead to a coma.

3. hypoglycemia: An abnormally low level of glucose in the blood. This condition can lead to a low-blood-sugar reaction. If your blood sugar level gets too low, you can act abnormally or pass out.

4. regular insulin: A short-acting insulin

5. lantus: A twenty-four-hour, long-acting insulin.

6. sliding-scale insulin: A set of instructions for administrating insulin doses based on specific blood-glucose readings.

You have to try not to miss any appointments with your doctor. If you do have to miss one, reschedule it as soon as possible. These appointments are very important to our survival. We cannot go two years without seeing a doctor, whatever his specialty is. Don't do as I did and go twenty-six years without seeing a foot doctor. That's right, twenty-six years, until I went in 2009 when I got a diabetic ulcer on my Achilles tendon. General practitioner, foot doctor, and eye doctor appointments are very important to us. It's up to us to keep the appointments. It is hard to predict how your body is going to handle insulin, so a doctor's guidance is crucial.

Diabetes can be different from day to day. You might be taking a certain amount of long-acting insulin, and everything seems to be working well. Then all of a sudden, one day your blood sugar starts running either extremely high or extremely low. This is something that just happens. Why? I don't know. Blood testing will help determine these things. If we make any long-acting insulin changes, they should should be made one unit at a time. Dealing with this disease can be quite a challenge.

At times, with all the things there are to deal with, it's easy to suffer from depression. Have I felt depressed at times? Yes. But the fact that I am able to tell this story proves that I'm a living miracle. It is a miracle just to be living.

About the Author

Ethereal T. Henry Jr.
henryetherealjr@yahoo.com

I grew up in East St. Louis, Illinois. I currently live in St. Louis, Missouri. I have lived in St. Louis, Missouri, for thirty-one years. I have never changed doctors. I have been an insulin-dependent diabetic since April 1983. I enjoy the computer, fishing, and reading. My prescription for blood strips says "test eight times daily." I have tried to learn everything I could about sugar diabetes since I learned about the complications that can occur. My wife has really helped me deal with this disease over the years. It's good to talk about this disease. Tell people what you are trying to accomplish. They won't know what you are going through unless you tell them. Being silent and minding your own business is not a good policy. What I can tell somebody might help someone else. How we do that is by talking. What am I trying to accomplish? Great A1c test readings between 7.9 and 6.0. Dealing with this disease has been quite a journey. I have had car mishaps that I haven't even mentioned. This is the main reason I blood test while I'm driving. I have to do what works best for me. It only takes about ten seconds or so. I hope that by reading this, you will be able to live a happier life.